30-DAY DIABETIC COOKBOOK MEAL PLAN FOR BEGINNERS

A Comprehensive 30-Day Diabetic Cookbook Meal Plan to Kickstart Your Journey

Dr Lily Morgan

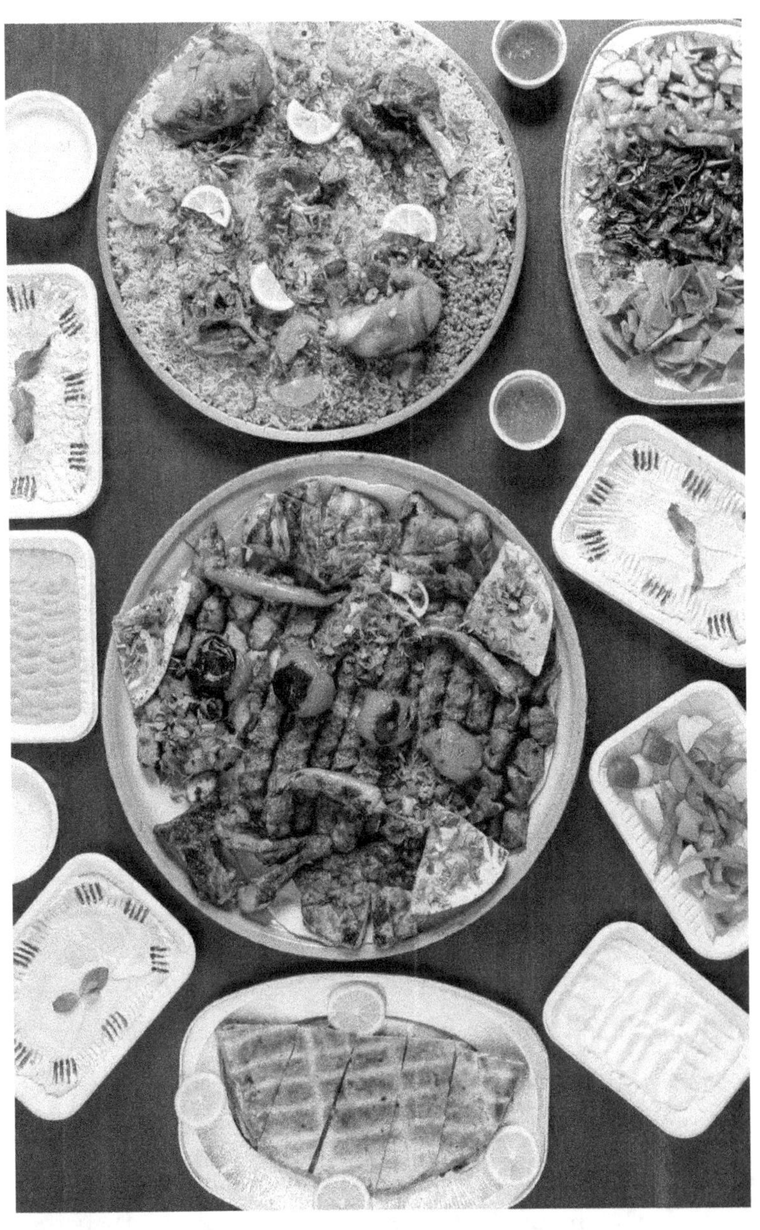

TABLE OF CONTENTS

Chapter 5: Snacks and Appetizers 78

Chapter 6: Desserts 90

INTRODUCTION

In today's fast-paced world, where lifestyle diseases are on the rise, it becomes increasingly important to prioritize our health and well-being. One such prevalent health condition is diabetes, a chronic metabolic disorder characterized by high blood sugar levels. Managing diabetes requires careful attention to one's diet, and that's where this "30-Day Diabetic Cookbook Meal Plan for Beginners" comes in.

This comprehensive meal plan has been specially curated to cater to individuals who are new to managing diabetes. Whether you have recently been diagnosed with diabetes or are looking for a fresh start on your journey towards a healthier lifestyle, this cookbook is designed to make your transition easier and more enjoyable.

Understanding Diabetes and Diet Management

Diabetes is a chronic condition that affects millions of people worldwide. It is characterized by the body's inability to properly regulate blood sugar levels, leading to elevated glucose levels in the bloodstream. Proper management of diabetes is crucial to prevent complications and maintain overall health.

In this section, we will explore the different types of diabetes, such as Type 1 and Type 2 diabetes, as well as gestational diabetes. We will discuss the underlying causes, symptoms, and the impact of diet on diabetes management. Understanding the relationship between carbohydrates, insulin, and blood sugar levels will provide a solid foundation for designing an effective meal plan.

Importance of a Balanced Diabetic Meal Plan

A balanced diabetic meal plan plays a pivotal role in maintaining stable blood sugar levels and promoting overall well-being. A well-designed meal plan ensures that individuals with diabetes receive the necessary nutrients while managing their carbohydrate intake.

In this section, we will explore the key components of a balanced diabetic meal plan. We will discuss the importance of portion control, the significance of macronutrients (carbohydrates, proteins, and fats) in managing diabetes, and the role of fiber in stabilizing blood sugar levels. Additionally, we will delve into the concept of glycemic index and how it can guide food choices to support optimal diabetes management.

Tips for Successful Meal Planning

Meal planning is a fundamental aspect of a diabetic lifestyle. It helps individuals with diabetes maintain control over their diet, making it easier to manage blood sugar levels and make healthier food choices. This section will provide practical tips and strategies for successful meal planning.

We will explore the importance of grocery shopping with a plan, reading food labels to identify hidden sugars, and incorporating a variety of foods to ensure a well-rounded diet. Additionally, we will discuss the significance of meal prepping and how it can save time and effort throughout the week. We will also touch upon mindful eating practices and the importance of staying hydrated.

Furthermore, we will address the challenges that beginners may face when adopting a diabetic meal plan and offer solutions to overcome them. Tips for dining out, navigating social gatherings, and managing cravings will empower individuals to make informed decisions and stay on track with their diabetic meal plan.

Chapter 1: 30-Day Meal Plan

Week 1:

Day 1:

Breakfast: Vegetable Omelet with Spinach and Bell Peppers

Lunch: Grilled Chicken and Vegetable Salad with Balsamic Vinaigrette

Dinner: Baked Lemon Herb Salmon with Roasted Vegetables

Snack: Guacamole with Veggie Sticks

Dessert: Berry Chia Seed Jam

Smoothie: Green Detox Smoothie

Day 2:

Breakfast: Avocado and Tomato Breakfast Salad

Lunch: Turkey and Avocado Lettuce Wraps

Dinner: Grilled Chicken with Cauliflower Rice

Snack: Caprese Skewers with Balsamic Glaze

Dessert: Baked Apples with Cinnamon and Walnuts

Smoothie: Blueberry and Spinach Smoothie

Day 3:

Breakfast: Cinnamon Apple Overnight Oats

Lunch: Quinoa and Black Bean Salad with Lime Dressing

Dinner: Ratatouille with Quinoa

Snack: Greek Yogurt and Berry Popsicles

Dessert: Chocolate Avocado Mousse

Smoothie: Mango and Turmeric Smoothie

Day 4:

Breakfast: Greek Yogurt Parfait with Berries and Nuts

Lunch: Salmon and Vegetable Stir-Fry

Dinner: Turkey Meatballs in Tomato Sauce

Snack: Oven-Baked Sweet Potato Fries

Dessert: Greek Yogurt and Mixed Berry Parfait

Smoothie: Strawberry and Kale Smoothie

Day 5:

Breakfast: Zucchini and Feta Muffins

Lunch: Mediterranean Chickpea Salad

Dinner: Beef and Vegetable Stir-Fry

Snack: Cucumber and Hummus Bites

Dessert: Sugar-Free Blueberry Cheesecake Bites

Smoothie: Avocado and Coconut Smoothie

Day 6:

Breakfast: Quinoa Breakfast Bowl with Berries and Almonds

Lunch: Spinach and Goat Cheese Stuffed Chicken Breast

Dinner: Stuffed Portobello Mushrooms with Quinoa and Spinach

Snack: Roasted Chickpeas with Chili and Lime

Dessert: Almond Flour Chocolate Chip Cookies

Smoothie: Pineapple and Ginger Smoothie

Day 7:

Breakfast: Spinach and Mushroom Frittata

Lunch: Vegetable and Lentil Soup

Dinner: Lemon Garlic Shrimp Skewers with Zucchini Noodles

Snack: Zucchini Chips with Garlic and Parmesan

Dessert: Coconut and Lime Energy Balls

Smoothie: Berry Blast Smoothie

Week 2:

Day 8:

Breakfast: Whole Wheat Pancakes with Sugar-Free Blueberry Compote

Lunch: Tuna Salad Lettuce Wraps

Dinner: Lentil Curry with Brown Rice

Snack: Smoked Salmon Cucumber Rolls

Dessert: Pumpkin Spice Chia Pudding

Smoothie: Peanut Butter and Banana Smoothie

Day 9:

Breakfast: Smoked Salmon and Cream Cheese Wrap

Lunch: Shrimp and Quinoa Stir-Fry

Dinner: Chicken and Vegetable Kebabs with Greek Yogurt Sauce

Snack: Turkey and Cheese Roll-Ups

Dessert: Peanut Butter and Banana Ice Cream

Smoothie: Chocolate and Almond Smoothie

Day 10:

Breakfast: Chia Seed Pudding with Mixed Berries

Lunch: Mexican-Style Stuffed Bell Peppers

Dinner: Spaghetti Squash with Turkey Bolognese

Snack: Edamame with Sea Salt

Dessert: Strawberry Frozen Yogurt Bark

Smoothie: Tropical Green Smoothie

Day 11:

Breakfast: Scrambled Tofu with Vegetables

Lunch: Greek Salad with Grilled Shrimp

Dinner: Teriyaki Tofu Stir-Fry with Broccoli and Brown Rice

Snack: Stuffed Mini Bell Peppers with Cream Cheese

Dessert: Raspberry and Almond Flour Cake

Smoothie: Coffee and Walnut Smoothie

Day 12:

Breakfast: Vegetable Omelet with Spinach and Bell Peppers

Lunch: Grilled Chicken and Vegetable Salad with Balsamic Vinaigrette

Dinner: Baked Lemon Herb Salmon with Roasted Vegetables

Snack: Guacamole with Veggie Sticks

Dessert: Berry Chia Seed Jam

Smoothie: Green Detox Smoothie

Day 13:

Breakfast: Avocado and Tomato Breakfast Salad

Lunch: Turkey and Avocado Lettuce Wraps

Dinner: Grilled Chicken with Cauliflower Rice

Snack: Caprese Skewers with Balsamic Glaze

Dessert: Baked Apples with Cinnamon and Walnuts

Smoothie: Blueberry and Spinach Smoothie

Day 14:

Breakfast: Cinnamon Apple Overnight Oats

Lunch: Quinoa and Black Bean Salad with Lime Dressing

Dinner: Ratatouille with Quinoa

Snack: Greek Yogurt and Berry Popsicles

Dessert: Chocolate Avocado Mousse

Smoothie: Mango and Turmeric Smoothie

Week 3:

Day 15:

Breakfast: Greek Yogurt Parfait with Berries and Nuts

Lunch: Salmon and Vegetable Stir-Fry

Dinner: Turkey Meatballs in Tomato Sauce

Snack: Oven-Baked Sweet Potato Fries

Dessert: Greek Yogurt and Mixed Berry Parfait

Smoothie: Strawberry and Kale Smoothie

Day 16:

Breakfast: Zucchini and Feta Muffins

Lunch: Mediterranean Chickpea Salad

Dinner: Beef and Vegetable Stir-Fry

Snack: Cucumber and Hummus Bites

Dessert: Sugar-Free Blueberry Cheesecake Bites

Smoothie: Avocado and Coconut Smoothie

Day 17:

Breakfast: Quinoa Breakfast Bowl with Berries and Almonds

Lunch: Spinach and Goat Cheese Stuffed Chicken Breast

Dinner: Stuffed Portobello Mushrooms with Quinoa and Spinach

Snack: Roasted Chickpeas with Chili and Lime

Dessert: Almond Flour Chocolate Chip Cookies

Smoothie: Pineapple and Ginger Smoothie

Day 18:

Breakfast: Spinach and Mushroom Frittata

Lunch: Vegetable and Lentil Soup

Dinner: Lemon Garlic Shrimp Skewers with Zucchini Noodles

Snack: Zucchini Chips with Garlic and Parmesan

Dessert: Coconut and Lime Energy Balls

Smoothie: Berry Blast Smoothie

Day 19:

Breakfast: Whole Wheat Pancakes with Sugar-Free Blueberry Compote

Lunch: Tuna Salad Lettuce Wraps

Dinner: Lentil Curry with Brown Rice

Snack: Smoked Salmon Cucumber Rolls

Dessert: Pumpkin Spice Chia Pudding

Smoothie: Peanut Butter and Banana Smoothie

Day 20:

Breakfast: Smoked Salmon and Cream Cheese Wrap

Lunch: Shrimp and Quinoa Stir-Fry

Dinner: Chicken and Vegetable Kebabs with Greek Yogurt Sauce

Snack: Turkey and Cheese Roll-Ups

Dessert: Peanut Butter and Banana Ice Cream

Smoothie: Chocolate and Almond Smoothie

Day 21:

Breakfast: Chia Seed Pudding with Mixed Berries

Lunch: Mexican-Style Stuffed Bell Peppers

Dinner: Spaghetti Squash with Turkey Bolognese

Snack: Edamame with Sea Salt

Dessert: Strawberry Frozen Yogurt Bark

Smoothie: Tropical Green Smoothie

Week 4:

Day 22:

Breakfast: Scrambled Tofu with Vegetables

Lunch: Greek Salad with Grilled Shrimp

Dinner: Teriyaki Tofu Stir-Fry with Broccoli and Brown Rice

Snack: Stuffed Mini Bell Peppers with Cream Cheese

Dessert: Raspberry and Almond Flour Cake

Smoothie: Coffee and Walnut Smoothie

Day 23:

Breakfast: Vegetable Omelet with Spinach and Bell Peppers

Lunch: Grilled Chicken and Vegetable Salad with Balsamic Vinaigrette

Dinner: Baked Lemon Herb Salmon with Roasted Vegetables

Snack: Guacamole with Veggie Sticks

Dessert: Berry Chia Seed Jam

Smoothie: Green Detox Smoothie

Day 24:

Breakfast: Avocado and Tomato Breakfast Salad

Lunch: Turkey and Avocado Lettuce Wraps

Dinner: Grilled Chicken with Cauliflower Rice

Snack: Caprese Skewers with Balsamic Glaze

Dessert: Baked Apples with Cinnamon and Walnuts

Smoothie: Blueberry and Spinach Smoothie

Day 25:

Breakfast: Cinnamon Apple Overnight Oats

Lunch: Quinoa and Black Bean Salad with Lime Dressing

Dinner: Ratatouille with Quinoa

Snack: Greek Yogurt and Berry Popsicles

Dessert: Chocolate Avocado Mousse

Smoothie: Mango and Turmeric Smoothie

Day 26:

Breakfast: Greek Yogurt Parfait with Berries and Nuts

Lunch: Salmon and Vegetable Stir-Fry

Dinner: Turkey Meatballs in Tomato Sauce

Snack: Oven-Baked Sweet Potato Fries

Dessert: Greek Yogurt and Mixed Berry Parfait

Smoothie: Strawberry and Kale Smoothie

Day 27:

Breakfast: Zucchini and Feta Muffins

Lunch: Mediterranean Chickpea Salad

Dinner: Beef and Vegetable Stir-Fry

Snack: Cucumber and Hummus Bites

Dessert: Sugar-Free Blueberry Cheesecake Bites

Smoothie: Avocado and Coconut Smoothie

Day 28:

Breakfast: Quinoa Breakfast Bowl with Berries and Almonds

Lunch: Spinach and Goat Cheese Stuffed Chicken Breast

Dinner: Stuffed Portobello Mushrooms with Quinoa and Spinach

Snack: Roasted Chickpeas with Chili and Lime

Dessert: Almond Flour Chocolate Chip Cookies

Smoothie: Pineapple and Ginger Smoothie

Day 29:

Breakfast: Spinach and Mushroom Frittata

Lunch: Vegetable and Lentil Soup

Dinner: Lemon Garlic Shrimp Skewers with Zucchini Noodles

Snack: Zucchini Chips with Garlic and Parmesan

Dessert: Coconut and Lime Energy Balls

Smoothie: Berry Blast Smoothie

Day 30:

Breakfast: Scrambled Tofu with Vegetables

Lunch: Greek Salad with Grilled Shrimp

Dinner: Teriyaki Tofu Stir-Fry with Broccoli and Brown Rice

Snack: Stuffed Mini Bell Peppers with Cream Cheese

Dessert: Raspberry and Almond Flour Cake

Smoothie: Coffee and Walnut Smoothie

Chapter 2: Breakfast Recipes

In this chapter, we will explore delicious and nutritious breakfast recipes that are perfect for starting your day on a healthy note. These recipes are designed to provide you with energy and essential nutrients while keeping your blood sugar levels stable. Let's dive in!

Vegetable Omelet with Spinach and Bell Peppers

Ingredients:

- 2 eggs
- 1 tablespoon olive oil
- 1 cup fresh spinach, chopped
- 1/4 cup bell peppers, diced
- Salt and pepper to taste

Instructions:

1. Heat the olive oil in a non-stick skillet over medium heat.

2. Add the bell peppers and sauté for 2-3 minutes until they start to soften.

3. Add the chopped spinach and cook for another 2 minutes until wilted.

4. In a bowl, beat the eggs and season with salt and pepper.

5. Pour the beaten eggs over the vegetables in the skillet.

6. Cook for 2-3 minutes or until the edges of the omelet start to set.

7. Carefully flip the omelet and cook for another 2-3 minutes until cooked through.

8. Slide the omelet onto a plate and serve hot.

Avocado and Tomato Breakfast Salad

Ingredients:

- 1 ripe avocado, diced
- 1 cup cherry tomatoes, halved
- 1/4 cup red onion, thinly sliced
- 1 tablespoon fresh lemon juice
- 1 tablespoon extra virgin olive oil

- Salt and pepper to taste
- Fresh basil leaves for garnish

Instructions:

1. In a bowl, combine the diced avocado, cherry tomatoes, and sliced red onion.
2. In a small separate bowl, whisk together the lemon juice and olive oil.
3. Drizzle the dressing over the avocado and tomato mixture.
4. Season with salt and pepper and gently toss to combine.
5. Garnish with fresh basil leaves and serve as a refreshing breakfast salad.

Cinnamon Apple Overnight Oats

Ingredients:

- 1/2 cup rolled oats
- 1/2 cup unsweetened almond milk
- 1/4 cup plain Greek yogurt
- 1 tablespoon chia seeds
- 1 tablespoon maple syrup

- 1/2 teaspoon ground cinnamon
- 1 apple, diced
- Crushed nuts for topping (optional)

Instructions:

1. In a mason jar or airtight container, combine the rolled oats, almond milk, Greek yogurt, chia seeds, maple syrup, and ground cinnamon.
2. Stir well to ensure all the ingredients are thoroughly combined.
3. Add the diced apple to the mixture and stir again.
4. Seal the container and refrigerate overnight or for at least 6 hours.
5. In the morning, give the oats a good stir and top with crushed nuts if desired.
6. Enjoy your creamy and flavorful cinnamon apple overnight oats.

Greek Yogurt Parfait with Berries and Nuts

Ingredients:

- 1 cup plain Greek yogurt

- 1/4 cup mixed berries (strawberries, blueberries, raspberries)
- 2 tablespoons chopped nuts (almonds, walnuts, or pistachios)
- 1 tablespoon honey or agave syrup

Instructions:

1. In a glass or bowl, layer the Greek yogurt, mixed berries, and chopped nuts.
2. Drizzle honey or agave syrup over the layers.
3. Repeat the layers until all the ingredients are used.
4. Finish with a sprinkle of nuts on top for added crunch.
5. Serve the Greek yogurt parfait immediately and enjoy the creamy and fruity goodness.

Zucchini and Feta Muffins

Ingredients:

- 1 cup grated zucchini
- 1/2 cup crumbled feta cheese
- 1/4 cup chopped fresh dill
- 2 cups whole wheat flour

- 1 teaspoon baking powder
- 1/2 teaspoon baking soda
- 1/2 teaspoon salt
- 1/4 teaspoon black pepper
- 2 eggs
- 1/2 cup plain Greek yogurt
- 1/4 cup olive oil

Instructions:

1. Preheat the oven to 350°F (175°C). Grease or line a muffin tin with paper liners.
2. In a large bowl, combine the grated zucchini, crumbled feta cheese, and chopped fresh dill.
3. In a separate bowl, whisk together the whole wheat flour, baking powder, baking soda, salt, and black pepper.
4. In another bowl, beat the eggs and then add the Greek yogurt and olive oil. Mix well.
5. Pour the wet ingredients into the bowl with the zucchini mixture and stir until combined.

6. Gradually add the dry ingredients to the zucchini mixture and stir until just combined. Do not overmix.

7. Spoon the batter into the prepared muffin tin, filling each cup about two-thirds full.

8. Bake for 18-20 minutes or until a toothpick inserted into the center of a muffin comes out clean.

9. Remove from the oven and allow the muffins to cool for a few minutes before transferring them to a wire rack to cool completely.

Quinoa Breakfast Bowl with Berries and Almonds

Ingredients:

- 1/2 cup cooked quinoa
- 1/4 cup mixed berries (strawberries, blueberries, raspberries)
- 2 tablespoons sliced almonds
- 1 tablespoon honey or maple syrup
- 1/4 teaspoon vanilla extract
- Pinch of cinnamon

Instructions:

1. In a bowl, combine the cooked quinoa, mixed berries, and sliced almonds.

2. Drizzle honey or maple syrup over the mixture.

3. Add the vanilla extract and a pinch of cinnamon.

4. Stir gently to combine all the ingredients.

5. Allow the flavors to meld for a few minutes before enjoying your nutritious quinoa breakfast bowl.

Spinach and Mushroom Frittata

Ingredients:

- 4 eggs
- 1/4 cup milk (dairy or plant-based)
- 1 cup fresh spinach leaves
- 1/2 cup sliced mushrooms
- 1/4 cup diced onion
- 1 clove garlic, minced
- 1 tablespoon olive oil
- Salt and pepper to taste
- Grated Parmesan cheese for topping (optional)

Instructions:

1. Preheat the oven to 350°F (175°C).

2. In a bowl, whisk together the eggs and milk. Set aside.

3. Heat the olive oil in an oven-safe skillet over medium heat.

4. Add the diced onion and minced garlic, and sauté until fragrant and slightly softened.

5. Add the sliced mushrooms and cook until they release their moisture and start to brown.

6. Stir in the fresh spinach leaves and cook until wilted.

7. Season the mixture with salt and pepper.

8. Pour the egg mixture over the vegetables in the skillet.

9. Cook for a few minutes until the edges start to set.

10. Sprinkle grated Parmesan cheese on top, if desired.

11. Transfer the skillet to the preheated oven and bake for 12-15 minutes or until the frittata is set in the center.

12. Remove from the ovenand let it cool for a few minutes before slicing and serving.

Whole Wheat Pancakes with Sugar-Free Blueberry Compote

Ingredients:

For the pancakes:

- 1 cup whole wheat flour
- 1 tablespoon baking powder
- 1/4 teaspoon salt
- 1 tablespoon honey or maple syrup
- 1 cup unsweetened almond milk (or any preferred milk)
- 1 egg
- 1 tablespoon melted coconut oil

For the blueberry compote:

- 1 cup fresh or frozen blueberries
- 2 tablespoons water
- 1 tablespoon lemon juice
- 1 tablespoon honey or a natural sugar substitute

Instructions:

For the pancakes:

1. In a large bowl, whisk together the whole wheat flour, baking powder, and salt.

2. In a separate bowl, whisk together the honey or maple syrup, almond milk, egg, and melted coconut oil.

3. Pour the wet ingredients into the bowl with the dry ingredients and stir until just combined. The batter may have some lumps, but that's okay.

4. Heat a non-stick skillet or griddle over medium heat and lightly grease with cooking spray or a small amount of coconut oil.

5. Pour 1/4 cup of the pancake batter onto the skillet for each pancake.

6. Cook until bubbles form on the surface of the pancake, then flip and cook for another 1-2 minutes until golden brown.

7. Repeat with the remaining batter, adding more oil if necessary.

8. Serve the whole wheat pancakes warm with the sugar-free blueberry compote.

For the blueberry compote:

1. In a small saucepan, combine the blueberries, water, lemon juice, and honey or sugar substitute.

2. Bring the mixture to a boil over medium heat, then reduce the heat to low and simmer for 8-10 minutes, stirring occasionally, until the blueberries break down and the compote thickens slightly.

3. Remove from heat and let it cool for a few minutes.

4. Use the compote as a topping for the whole wheat pancakes.

Smoked Salmon and Cream Cheese Wrap

Ingredients:

- 1 whole wheat tortilla or wrap
- 2 ounces smoked salmon
- 2 tablespoons cream cheese
- 1/4 cup baby spinach leaves
- 1/4 cup sliced cucumber
- Fresh dill for garnish

Instructions:

1. Lay the whole wheat tortilla or wrap on a clean surface.

2. Spread the cream cheese evenly over the tortilla.

3. Place the smoked salmon on top of the cream cheese.

4. Add the baby spinach leaves and sliced cucumber.

5. Garnish with fresh dill.

6. Roll the tortilla tightly into a wrap.

7. Slice the wrap in half if desired, and serve.

Chia Seed Pudding with Mixed Berries

Ingredients:

- 1/4 cup chia seeds
- 1 cup unsweetened almond milk (or any preferred milk)
- 1 tablespoon honey or maple syrup
- 1/2 teaspoon vanilla extract
- 1/2 cup mixed berries (strawberries, blueberries, raspberries)
- Crushed nuts for topping (optional)

Instructions:

1. In a bowl or jar, combine the chia seeds, almond milk, honey or maple syrup, and vanilla extract.

2. Stir well to ensure the chia seeds are evenly distributed and not clumping together.

3. Cover the bowl or jar and refrigerate overnight or for at least 4 hours, allowing the chia seeds to absorb the liquid and form a pudding-like consistency.

4. Before serving, give the chia seed pudding a good stir to break up any clumps.

5. Top the pudding with mixed berries and crushed nuts for added flavor and texture.

6. Enjoy the creamy and nutrient-packed chia seed pudding for a satisfying breakfast.

Scrambled Tofu with Vegetables

Ingredients:

- 1/2 block firm tofu, drained and crumbled
- 1/4 cup diced bell peppers
- 1/4 cup diced onions
- 1/4 cup sliced mushrooms

- 1 clove garlic, minced
- 1 tablespoon olive oil
- 1/2 teaspoon ground turmeric
- 1/4 teaspoon ground cumin
- Salt and pepper to taste
- Chopped fresh parsley for garnish

Instructions:

1. Heat the olive oil in a skillet over medium heat.
2. Add the diced bell peppers, onions, and sliced mushrooms to the skillet and sauté for 3-4 minutes until they start to soften.
3. Add the minced garlic and cook for an additional 1 minute until fragrant.
4. Crumble the tofu into the skillet and stir to combine with the vegetables.
5. Sprinkle the ground turmeric and ground cumin over the tofu mixture.
6. Season with salt and pepper to taste.
7. Cook for 4-5 minutes, stirring occasionally, until the tofu is heated through and lightly browned.

8. Remove from heat and garnish with chopped fresh parsley.

9. Serve the scrambled tofu with vegetables as a protein-rich breakfast option.

Chapter 3: Lunch Recipes

These lunch recipes provide a variety of flavors and ingredients to keep your diabetic meal plan interesting and satisfying. Enjoy these delicious and nutritious meals while managing your diabetes and promoting overall health and well-being.

Grilled Chicken and Vegetable Salad with Balsamic Vinaigrette

Ingredients:

- 2 boneless, skinless chicken breasts
- 2 cups mixed salad greens
- 1 cup cherry tomatoes, halved
- 1 cup cucumber, sliced
- 1/2 cup red onion, thinly sliced
- 1/4 cup feta cheese, crumbled
- 2 tablespoons balsamic vinegar
- 2 tablespoons olive oil
- 1 teaspoon Dijon mustard
- Salt and pepper to taste

Instructions:

1. Preheat the grill to medium-high heat.
2. Season the chicken breasts with salt and pepper.
3. Grill the chicken for 6-8 minutes per side until cooked through. Let it rest for a few minutes, then slice it into thin strips.
4. In a large salad bowl, combine the mixed greens, cherry tomatoes, cucumber, and red onion.
5. In a small bowl, whisk together the balsamic vinegar, olive oil, Dijon mustard, salt, and pepper to make the dressing.
6. Drizzle the dressing over the salad and toss to coat.
7. Divide the salad onto plates and top with grilled chicken slices.
8. Sprinkle the crumbled feta cheese over the salad.
9. Serve the grilled chicken and vegetable salad immediately.

Turkey and Avocado Lettuce Wraps

Ingredients:

- 1 pound ground turkey
- 1 tablespoon olive oil

- 2 cloves garlic, minced
- 1 teaspoon ground cumin
- 1/2 teaspoon chili powder
- 1/2 teaspoon paprika
- Salt and pepper to taste
- 1 avocado, diced
- 1/4 cup red onion, finely chopped
- 1/4 cup fresh cilantro, chopped
- Juice of 1 lime
- Lettuce leaves for wrapping

Instructions:

1. Heat the olive oil in a skillet over medium heat.
2. Add the minced garlic and cook for 1 minute until fragrant.
3. Add the ground turkey to the skillet and cook until browned and cooked through.
4. Stir in the ground cumin, chili powder, paprika, salt, and pepper. Cook for an additional 2-3 minutes.
5. In a bowl, combine the diced avocado, red onion, cilantro, and lime juice.

6. Place a spoonful of the turkey mixture onto each lettuce leaf.

7. Top with a spoonful of the avocado mixture.

8. Roll up the lettuce leaves to form wraps.

9. Serve the turkey and avocado lettuce wraps as a healthy and flavorful lunch option.

Quinoa and Black Bean Salad with Lime Dressing

Ingredients:

- 1 cup cooked quinoa
- 1 cup black beans, rinsed and drained
- 1 cup cherry tomatoes, halved
- 1 cup cucumber, diced
- 1/4 cup red onion, finely chopped
- 1/4 cup fresh cilantro, chopped
- 2 tablespoons lime juice
- 2 tablespoons olive oil
- 1 clove garlic, minced
- Salt and pepper to taste

Instructions:

1. In a large bowl, combine the cooked quinoa, black beans, cherry tomatoes, cucumber, red onion, and cilantro.
2. In a small bowl, whisk together the lime juice, olive oil, minced garlic, salt, and pepper to make the dressing.
3. Pour the dressing over the quinoa and black bean mixture and toss to coat.
4. Adjust the seasoning if needed.
5. Cover the bowl and refrigerate the salad for at least 30 minutes to allow the flavors to meld together.
6. Serve the quinoa and black bean salad as a refreshing and protein-packed lunch option.

Salmon and Vegetable Stir-Fry

Ingredients:

- 2 salmon fillets
- 2 tablespoons low-sodium soy sauce
- 1 tablespoon honey
- 1 tablespoon rice vinegar
- 1 tablespoon sesame oil

- 1 tablespoon cornstarch
- 2 tablespoons olive oil
- 2 cloves garlic, minced
- 1 tablespoon grated ginger
- 1 red bell pepper, thinly sliced
- 1 cup broccoli florets
- 1 cup snap peas
- 1 carrot, julienned
- 2 green onions, chopped
- Sesame seeds for garnish (optional)

Instructions:

1. In a small bowl, whisk together the soy sauce, honey, rice vinegar, sesame oil, and cornstarch to make the sauce. Set aside.
2. Season the salmon fillets with salt and pepper.
3. Heat the olive oil in a skillet over medium-high heat.
4. Add the salmon fillets, skin side down, and cook for 3-4 minutes until crispy.

5. Flip the salmon and cook for an additional 3-4 minutes until cooked through. Remove from the skillet and set aside.

6. In the same skillet, add the minced garlic and grated ginger. Cook for 1 minute until fragrant.

7. Add the sliced bell pepper, broccoli florets, snap peas, and julienned carrot to the skillet. Stir-fry for 4-5 minutes until the vegetables are crisp-tender.

8. Pour the sauce over the vegetables and cook for an additional 1-2 minutes until the sauce thickens.

9. Return the salmon fillets to the skillet and coat them with the sauce and vegetables.

10. Garnish with chopped green onions and sesame seeds, if desired.

11. Serve the salmon and vegetable stir-fry hot over steamed rice or quinoa.

Mediterranean Chickpea Salad

Ingredients:

- 2 cups cooked chickpeas
- 1 cup cherry tomatoes, halved
- 1 cup cucumber, diced

- 1/2 cup Kalamata olives, pitted and halved
- 1/4 cup red onion, thinly sliced
- 1/4 cup crumbled feta cheese
- 2 tablespoons fresh lemon juice
- 2 tablespoons extra virgin olive oil
- 1 clove garlic, minced
- 1 teaspoon dried oregano
- Salt and pepper to taste

Instructions:

1. In a large bowl, combine the cooked chickpeas, cherry tomatoes, cucumber, Kalamata olives, red onion, and crumbled feta cheese.
2. In a small bowl, whisk together the lemon juice, olive oil, minced garlic, dried oregano, salt, and pepper to make the dressing.
3. Pour the dressing over the chickpea mixture and toss to coat.
4. Adjust the seasoning if needed.
5. Cover the bowl and refrigerate the salad for at least 30 minutes to allow the flavors to meld together.

6. Serve the Mediterranean chickpea salad as a
    refreshing and protein-packed lunch option.

Spinach and Goat Cheese Stuffed Chicken Breast

Ingredients:

- 4 boneless, skinless chicken breasts
- 2 cups fresh spinach leaves
- 1/2 cup crumbled goat cheese
- 2 tablespoons olive oil
- 2 cloves garlic, minced
- Salt and pepper to taste

Instructions:

1. Preheat the oven to 375°F (190°C).
2. Using a sharp knife, cut a pocket into the side of
    each chicken breast.
3. Stuff each chickenbreast with a handful of fresh
    spinach leaves and a spoonful of crumbled goat
    cheese.
4. Season the chicken breasts with salt and pepper.

5. In an oven-safe skillet, heat the olive oil over medium-high heat.

6. Add the minced garlic and cook for 1 minute until fragrant.

7. Place the stuffed chicken breasts in the skillet and sear for 2-3 minutes on each side until browned.

8. Transfer the skillet to the preheated oven and bake for 15-20 minutes or until the chicken is cooked through and the cheese is melted.

9. Remove the skillet from the oven and let the chicken rest for a few minutes before serving.

10. Slice the spinach and goat cheese stuffed chicken breasts and serve with a side of steamed vegetables or a fresh salad.

Vegetable and Lentil Soup

Ingredients:

- 1 cup dried lentils
- 1 tablespoon olive oil
- 1 onion, chopped
- 2 carrots, diced
- 2 celery stalks, diced

- 2 cloves garlic, minced
- 1 teaspoon ground cumin
- 1 teaspoon dried thyme
- 4 cups low-sodium vegetable broth
- 2 cups water
- 2 cups chopped tomatoes
- 2 cups chopped kale
- Salt and pepper to taste

Instructions:

1. Rinse the dried lentils under cold water and set aside.
2. In a large pot, heat the olive oil over medium heat.
3. Add the chopped onion, carrots, and celery to the pot. Cook for 5 minutes until the vegetables start to soften.
4. Add the minced garlic, ground cumin, and dried thyme. Cook for 1 minute until fragrant.
5. Add the rinsed lentils, vegetable broth, water, chopped tomatoes, and chopped kale to the pot.
6. Season with salt and pepper to taste.

7. Bring the soup to a boil, then reduce the heat and simmer for 30-40 minutes until the lentils are tender.

8. Adjust the seasoning if needed.

9. Serve the vegetable and lentil soup hot, and enjoy a comforting and nutritious lunch.

Tuna Salad Lettuce Wraps

Ingredients:

- 2 cans tuna, drained
- 1/4 cup Greek yogurt
- 2 tablespoons mayonnaise
- 1 celery stalk, finely chopped
- 1/4 cup red onion, finely chopped
- 2 tablespoons fresh parsley, chopped
- 1 tablespoon lemon juice
- Salt and pepper to taste
- Lettuce leaves for wrapping

Instructions:

1. In a bowl, combine the drained tuna, Greek yogurt, mayonnaise, finely chopped celery, finely chopped

red onion, chopped fresh parsley, lemon juice, salt, and pepper.

2. Stir well until all the ingredients are evenly combined.

3. Place a spoonful of the tuna salad mixture onto each lettuce leaf.

4. Roll up the lettuce leaves to form wraps.

5. Serve the tuna salad lettuce wraps as a light and protein-rich lunch option.

Shrimp and Quinoa Stir-Fry

Ingredients:

- 1 cup cooked quinoa
- 1 pound shrimp, peeled and deveined
- 2 tablespoons soy sauce
- 1 tablespoon honey
- 1 tablespoon sesame oil
- 1 tablespoon olive oil
- 1 red bell pepper, thinly sliced
- 1 cup snap peas
- 1 carrot, julienned
- 2 cloves garlic, minced

- 1 tablespoon grated ginger

- 2 green onions, chopped

- Sesame seeds for garnish (optional)

Instructions:

1. In a small bowl, whisk together the soy sauce, honey, and sesame oil to make the sauce. Set aside.

2. In a large skillet, heat the olive oil over medium-high heat.

3. Add the shrimp to the skillet and cook for 2-3 minutes until pink and cooked through. Remove the shrimp from the skillet and set aside.

4. In the same skillet, add the red bell pepper, snap peas, julienned carrot, minced garlic, and grated ginger. Stir-fry for 3-4 minutes until the vegetables are crisp-tender.

5. Return the cooked shrimp to the skillet and pour the sauce over the shrimp and vegetables.

6. Cook for an additional 1-2 minutes until the sauce is heated through.

7. Stir in the cooked quinoa and chopped green onions.

8. Garnish with sesame seeds, if desired.

9. Serve the shrimp and quinoa stir-fry hot as a flavorful and nutritious lunch option.

Mexican-Style Stuffed Bell Peppers

Ingredients:

- 4 bell peppers (any color)
- 1 tablespoon olive oil
- 1 onion, chopped
- 2 cloves garlic, minced
- 1 pound ground turkey or beef
- 1 cup cooked brown rice
- 1 cup black beans, rinsed and drained
- 1 cup corn kernels
- 1 cup diced tomatoes
- 1 teaspoon chili powder
- 1/2 teaspoon ground cumin
- 1/2 teaspoon paprika
- Salt and pepper to taste
- 1/2 cup shredded cheddar cheese (optional)
- Fresh cilantro for garnish (optional)

Instructions:

1. Preheat the oven to 375°F (190°C).
2. Cut the tops off the bell peppers and remove the seeds and membranes. Set aside.
3. Heat the olive oil in a skillet over medium heat.
4. Add the chopped onion and minced garlic to the skillet and cook for 5 minutes until softened.
5. Add the ground turkey or beef to the skillet and cook until browned and cooked through.
6. Stir in the cooked brown rice, black beans, corn kernels, diced tomatoes, chili powder, ground cumin, paprika, salt, and pepper. Cook for an additional 2-3 minutes to heat through and combine the flavors.
7. Spoon the filling into the hollowed-out bell peppers.
8. If desired, sprinkle shredded cheddar cheese over the top of each stuffed bell pepper.
9. Place the stuffed bell peppers in a baking dish and cover with foil.
10. Bake for 25-30 minutes until the bell peppers are tender and the filling is heated through.

11. Remove from the oven and garnish with fresh cilantro, if desired.

12. Serve the Mexican-style stuffed bell peppers as a delicious and satisfying lunch option.

Greek Salad with Grilled Shrimp

Ingredients:

- 1 pound shrimp, peeled and deveined
- 2 tablespoons olive oil
- 2 tablespoons lemon juice
- 2 cloves garlic, minced
- 1 teaspoon dried oregano
- Salt and pepper to taste
- 4 cups mixed salad greens
- 1 cup cherry tomatoes, halved
- 1 cucumber, sliced
- 1/2 cup Kalamata olives, pitted
- 1/2 cup crumbled feta cheese
- 1/4 cup red onion, thinly sliced
- 2 tablespoons fresh lemon juice
- 2 tablespoons extra virgin olive oil
- Salt and pepper to taste

Instructions:

1. In a bowl, combine the shrimp, olive oil, lemon juice, minced garlic, dried oregano, salt, and pepper. Toss to coat the shrimp evenly.
2. Preheat thegrill or grill pan over medium-high heat.
3. Thread the marinated shrimp onto skewers.
4. Grill the shrimp for 2-3 minutes per side until cooked through and slightly charred.
5. Remove the shrimp from the skewers and set aside.
6. In a large salad bowl, combine the mixed salad greens, cherry tomatoes, cucumber slices, Kalamata olives, crumbled feta cheese, and thinly sliced red onion.
7. In a small bowl, whisk together the fresh lemon juice, extra virgin olive oil, salt, and pepper to make the dressing.
8. Drizzle the dressing over the salad and toss to coat.
9. Divide the salad onto plates and top with the grilled shrimp.
10. Serve the Greek salad with grilled shrimp as a light and refreshing lunch option.

Chapter 4: Dinner Recipes

Enjoy these delectable dinner recipes as part of your diabetic meal plan. Each dish is thoughtfully prepared to provide a healthy and flavorful option that will keep you satisfied and nourished.

Baked Lemon Herb Salmon with Roasted Vegetables

Ingredients:

- 4 salmon fillets
- 2 tablespoons fresh lemon juice
- 2 tablespoons olive oil
- 2 cloves garlic, minced
- 1 teaspoon dried thyme
- 1 teaspoon dried rosemary
- Salt and pepper, to taste
- 2 cups mixed vegetables (such as bell peppers, zucchini, and cherry tomatoes)
- Fresh parsley, for garnish

Instructions:

1. Preheat the oven to 400°F (200°C) and line a baking sheet with parchment paper.
2. In a small bowl, whisk together the lemon juice, olive oil, minced garlic, dried thyme, dried rosemary, salt, and pepper.
3. Place the salmon fillets on the prepared baking sheet and brush the lemon herb mixture over each fillet.
4. Arrange the mixed vegetables around the salmon on the baking sheet.
5. Bake in the preheated oven for 15-20 minutes, or until the salmon is cooked through and the vegetables are tender.
6. Garnish with fresh parsley and serve hot.

Grilled Chicken with Cauliflower Rice

Ingredients:

- 4 boneless, skinless chicken breasts
- 2 tablespoons olive oil
- 2 teaspoons paprika

- 1 teaspoon garlic powder
- 1 teaspoon dried oregano
- Salt and pepper, to taste
- 1 head cauliflower, riced
- 2 tablespoons chopped fresh parsley, for garnish

Instructions:

1. Preheat the grill to medium heat.
2. In a small bowl, combine the olive oil, paprika, garlic powder, dried oregano, salt, and pepper to make a marinade.
3. Rub the marinade evenly over the chicken breasts and let them marinate for at least 30 minutes.
4. Grill the chicken breasts for about 6-8 minutes per side, or until they are cooked through and reach an internal temperature of 165°F (74°C).
5. While the chicken is grilling, prepare the cauliflower rice by pulsing the cauliflower florets in a food processor until they resemble rice grains.
6. Heat a large skillet over medium heat and add the cauliflower rice. Sauté for 5-6 minutes, or until the cauliflower is tender.

7. Serve the grilled chicken over the cauliflower rice and garnish with chopped fresh parsley.

Ratatouille with Quinoa

Ingredients:

- 1 eggplant, diced
- 2 zucchini, diced
- 1 yellow bell pepper, diced
- 1 red bell pepper, diced
- 1 onion, diced
- 3 cloves garlic, minced
- 2 tablespoons olive oil
- 1 can (14 ounces) diced tomatoes
- 1 teaspoon dried basil
- 1 teaspoon dried oregano
- Salt and pepper, to taste
- 1 cup cooked quinoa
- Fresh basil leaves, for garnish

Instructions:

1. Heat the olive oil in a large pot or skillet over medium heat.

2. Add the diced eggplant, zucchini, bell peppers, onion, and minced garlic to the pot. Sauté for 5-6 minutes, or until the vegetables start to soften.

3. Stir in the diced tomatoes, dried basil, dried oregano, salt, and pepper. Reduce the heat to low and let the mixture simmer for 15-20 minutes, stirring occasionally.

4. While the ratatouille is simmering, cook the quinoa according to the package instructions.

5. Serve the ratatouille over a bed of cooked quinoa and garnish with fresh basil leaves.

Turkey Meatballs in Tomato Sauce

Ingredients:

- 1 pound ground turkey
- 1/2 cup whole wheat breadcrumbs
- 1/4 cup grated Parmesan cheese
- 1/4 cup chopped fresh parsley
- 1 egg
- 2 cloves garlic, minced
- 1 teaspoon dried oregano
- 1/2 teaspoon dried basil

- Salt and pepper, to taste
- 1 tablespoon olive oil
- 1 can (14 ounces) crushed tomatoes
- 1/2 teaspoon sugar (optional)
- Fresh basil leaves, for garnish

Instructions:

1. In a large bowl, combine the ground turkey, breadcrumbs, grated Parmesan cheese, chopped fresh parsley, egg, minced garlic, dried oregano, dried basil, salt, and pepper. Mix well until all the ingredients are evenly incorporated.
2. Shape the mixture into small meatballs, about 1 inch in diameter.
3. Heat the olive oil in a skillet over medium heat. Add the meatballs and cook for 5-6 minutes, turning occasionally, until they are browned on all sides.
4. Pour the crushed tomatoes into the skillet and add the sugar (if using). Stir to combine.
5. Reduce the heat to low, cover the skillet, and simmer for 15-20 minutes, or until the meatballs are cooked through.

6. Serve the turkey meatballs in tomato sauce,
    garnished with fresh basil leaves.

Beef and Vegetable Stir-Fry

Ingredients:

- 1 pound beef sirloin, thinly sliced
- 2 tablespoons low-sodium soy sauce
- 1 tablespoon hoisin sauce
- 1 tablespoon cornstarch
- 1 tablespoon olive oil
- 1 onion, sliced
- 1 red bell pepper, sliced
- 1 green bell pepper, sliced
- 1 cup snap peas
- 2 cloves garlic, minced
- 1 teaspoon grated fresh ginger
- 2 tablespoons low-sodium beef broth
- Salt and pepper, to taste
- Chopped green onions, for garnish

Instructions:

1. In a bowl, combine the sliced beef with soy sauce, hoisin sauce, and cornstarch. Mix well to coat the beef with the sauce mixture.
2. Heat the olive oil in a large skillet or wok over high heat.
3. Add the sliced onion, red bell pepper, green bell pepper, snap peas, minced garlic, and grated ginger to the skillet. Stir-fry for 3-4 minutes, or until the vegetables are crisp-tender.
4. Remove the vegetables from the skillet and set them aside.
5. In the same skillet, add the beef slices and stir-fry for 2-3 minutes, or until they are cooked to your desired level of doneness.
6. Return the cooked vegetables to the skillet and add the low-sodium beef broth. Season with salt and pepper to taste.
7. Cook for an additional 1-2 minutes, until the sauce has thickened slightly.
8. Garnish with chopped green onions and serve hot.

Stuffed Portobello Mushrooms with Quinoa and Spinach

Ingredients:

- 4 large Portobello mushrooms
- 1 cup cooked quinoa
- 1 cup chopped spinach
- 1/2 cup crumbled feta cheese
- 2 cloves garlic, minced
- 2 tablespoons olive oil
- 1 tablespoon balsamic vinegar
- Salt and pepper, to taste
- Fresh basil leaves, for garnish

Instructions:

1. Preheat the oven to 375°F (190°C) and line a baking sheet with parchment paper.
2. Remove the stems from the Portobello mushrooms and gently scrape out the gills using a spoon.
3. In a bowl, combine the cooked quinoa, chopped spinach, crumbled feta cheese, minced garlic, olive oil, balsamic vinegar, salt, and pepper. Mix well.

4. Spoon the quinoa and spinach mixture into the Portobello mushroom caps, dividing it evenly among them.

5. Place the stuffed mushrooms on the prepared baking sheet and bake in the preheated oven for 20-25 minutes, or until the mushrooms are tender and the filling is heated through.

6. Garnish with fresh basil leaves and serve warm.

Lemon Garlic Shrimp Skewers with Zucchini Noodles

Ingredients:

- 1 pound large shrimp, peeled and deveined
- Zest and juice of 1 lemon
- 3 cloves garlic, minced
- 2 tablespoons olive oil
- Salt and pepper, to taste
- 2 zucchini, spiralized into noodles
- Fresh parsley, for garnish

Instructions:

1. In a bowl, combine the peeled and deveined shrimp
    with the lemon zest, lemon juice, minced garlic,
    olive oil, salt, and pepper. Toss well to coat the
    shrimp in the marinade. Let it marinate for 15-20
    minutes.

2. Preheat a grill or grill pan over medium-high heat.

3. Thread the marinated shrimp onto skewers.

4. Grill the shrimp skewers for 2-3 minutes per side, or
    until they are pink and opaque.

5. While the shrimp are grilling, heat a skillet over
    medium heat and add the zucchini noodles. Sauté
    for 2-3 minutes, or until the noodles are just tender.

6. Serve the grilled lemon garlic shrimp skewers over
    a bed of sautéed zucchini noodles.

7. Garnish with fresh parsley and serve immediately.

Lentil Curry with Brown Rice

Ingredients:

- 1 cup dried green lentils
- 1 tablespoon olive oil
- 1 onion, diced
- 2 cloves garlic, minced

- 1 tablespoon grated fresh ginger

- 2 tablespoons curry powder

- 1 teaspoon ground cumin

- 1/2 teaspoon ground turmeric

- 1 can (14 ounces) diced tomatoes

- 1 can (14 ounces) coconut milk

- Salt and pepper, to taste

- Cooked brown rice, for serving

- Fresh cilantro leaves, for garnish

Instructions:

1. Rinse the dried green lentils under cold water and drain.

2. In a large pot, heat the olive oil over medium heat. Add the diced onion and sauté until it becomes translucent.

3. Add the minced garlic and grated ginger to the pot and cook for an additional minute.

4. Stir in the curry powder, ground cumin, and ground turmeric. Cook for 1 minute, stirring constantly to toast the spices.

5. Add the rinsed lentils, diced tomatoes (with their juice), and coconut milk to the pot. Stir well to combine.

6. Bring the mixture to a boil, then reduce the heat to low. Cover the pot and let the curry simmer for 30-40 minutes, or until the lentils are tender and cooked through.

7. Season the lentil curry with salt and pepper, to taste.

8. Serve the lentil curry over cooked brown rice and garnish with fresh cilantro leaves.

Chicken and Vegetable Kebabs with Greek Yogurt Sauce

Ingredients:

- 2 boneless, skinless chicken breasts, cut into chunks
- 1 red bell pepper, cut into chunks
- 1 yellow bell pepper, cut into chunks
- 1 zucchini, sliced
- 1 red onion, cut into chunks
- 2 tablespoons olive oil
- 1 teaspoon dried oregano
- 1/2 teaspoon dried thyme

- Salt and pepper, to taste

- Wooden or metal skewers

- 1 cup plain Greek yogurt

- 1 tablespoon lemon juice

- 1 clove garlic, minced

- 1 tablespoon chopped fresh dill

- Salt and pepper, to taste

Instructions:

1. Preheat the grill to medium heat.

2. In a bowl, combine the chicken chunks, red bell pepper chunks, yellow bell pepper chunks, sliced zucchini, red onion chunks, olive oil, dried oregano, dried thyme, salt, and pepper. Toss well to coat the chicken and vegetables in the marinade.

3. Thread the marinated chicken and vegetables onto skewers, alternating the ingredients.

4. Grill the chicken and vegetable kebabs for 10-12 minutes, turning occasionally, or until the chicken is cooked through and the vegetables are tender.

5. While the kebabs are grilling, prepare the Greek yogurt sauce by combining the plain Greek yogurt,

lemon juice, minced garlic, chopped fresh dill, salt, and pepper in a bowl. Mix well.

6. Serve the chicken and vegetable kebabs with the Greek yogurt sauce on the side.

Spaghetti Squash with Turkey Bolognese

Ingredients:

- 1 spaghetti squash
- 1 tablespoon olive oil
- 1 pound ground turkey
- 1 onion, diced
- 2 cloves garlic, minced
- 1 carrot, diced
- 1 celery stalk, diced
- 1 can (14 ounces) crushed tomatoes
- 1 tablespoon tomato paste
- 1 teaspoon dried basil
- 1 teaspoon dried oregano
- Salt and pepper, to taste
- Fresh basil leaves, for garnish
- Grated Parmesan cheese, for serving (optional)

Instructions:

1. Preheat the oven to 400°F (200°C).
2. Cut the spaghetti squash in half lengthwise and scoop out the seeds. Place the squash halves cut-side up on a baking sheet.
3. Drizzle the olive oil over the cut sides of the spaghetti squash and season with salt and pepper.
4. Bake the spaghetti squash in the preheated oven for 40-50 minutes, or until the flesh is tender and easily separates into spaghetti-like strands with a fork.
5. While the spaghetti squash is baking, heat a skillet over medium heat and add the ground turkey. Cook the turkey, breaking it up with a spoon, until it is browned and cooked through.
6. Add the diced onion, minced garlic, diced carrot, and diced celery to the skillet. Sauté for 5-6 minutes, or until the vegetables start to soften.
7. Stir in the crushed tomatoes, tomato paste, dried basil, dried oregano, salt, and pepper. Simmer the bolognese sauce for 10-15 minutes, stirring occasionally.

8. Once the spaghetti squash is cooked, use a fork to scrape the flesh into spaghetti-like strands.

9. Serve the spaghetti squash with the turkey bolognese sauce on top.

10. Garnish with fresh basil leaves andsprinkle with grated Parmesan cheese, if desired.

Teriyaki Tofu Stir-Fry with Broccoli and Brown Rice

Ingredients:

- 1 block (14 ounces) firm tofu, drained and cubed
- 1/4 cup low-sodium soy sauce
- 2 tablespoons honey or maple syrup
- 2 tablespoons rice vinegar
- 1 tablespoon sesame oil
- 2 cloves garlic, minced
- 1 teaspoon grated fresh ginger
- 1 tablespoon cornstarch
- 2 tablespoons water
- 2 tablespoons olive oil
- 2 cups broccoli florets
- 1 red bell pepper, sliced

- 1 carrot, sliced
- Cooked brown rice, for serving
- Toasted sesame seeds, for garnish

Instructions:

1. In a bowl, combine the cubed tofu, low-sodium soy sauce, honey or maple syrup, rice vinegar, sesame oil, minced garlic, and grated ginger. Toss gently to coat the tofu in the teriyaki sauce. Let it marinate for 15-20 minutes.
2. In a small bowl, whisk together the cornstarch and water to make a slurry. Set aside.
3. Heat the olive oil in a large skillet or wok over medium-high heat.
4. Add the marinated tofu to the skillet, reserving the marinade, and cook for 5-6 minutes, or until the tofu is golden brown and slightly crispy.
5. Remove the tofu from the skillet and set it aside.
6. In the same skillet, add the broccoli florets, sliced red bell pepper, and sliced carrot. Stir-fry for 4-5 minutes, or until the vegetables are tender-crisp.

7. Return the cooked tofu to the skillet with the vegetables.

8. Pour the reserved marinade over the tofu and vegetables. Cook for 1-2 minutes, or until the sauce thickens slightly.

9. Serve the teriyaki tofu stir-fry over cooked brown rice.

10. Garnish with toasted sesame seeds.

Chapter 5: Snacks and Appetizers

Enjoy these delicious and healthy snacks and appetizers

Guacamole with Veggie Sticks

Ingredients:

- 2 ripe avocados
- 1 small onion, finely diced
- 1 tomato, diced
- 1 jalapeno pepper, seeded and minced
- 1 lime, juiced
- 2 tablespoons fresh cilantro, chopped
- Salt and pepper, to taste
- Assorted veggie sticks (carrots, celery, bell peppers) for serving

Instructions:

1. Cut the avocados in half and remove the pits. Scoop the flesh into a bowl and mash it with a fork.

2. Add the diced onion, tomato, jalapeno pepper, lime juice, and chopped cilantro to the bowl with the mashed avocado. Mix well.

3. Season the guacamole with salt and pepper according to your taste preferences.

4. Serve the guacamole with a platter of assorted veggie sticks for dipping.

Caprese Skewers with Balsamic Glaze

Ingredients:

- Cherry tomatoes
- Fresh mozzarella balls
- Fresh basil leaves
- Balsamic glaze
- Wooden skewers

Instructions:

1. Thread one cherry tomato, followed by a fresh mozzarella ball, and then a fresh basil leaf onto each skewer.

2. Repeat the process until you have assembled all the skewers.

3. Arrange the caprese skewers on a serving platter.

4. Drizzle the skewers with balsamic glaze just before serving.

Greek Yogurt and Berry Popsicles

Ingredients:

- 1 cup Greek yogurt
- 1 cup mixed berries (strawberries, blueberries, raspberries)
- 2 tablespoons honey or maple syrup
- Popsicle molds

Instructions:

1. In a blender, combine the Greek yogurt, mixed berries, and honey or maple syrup. Blend until smooth.

2. Pour the mixture into popsicle molds, leaving a little space at the top for expansion.

3. Insert popsicle sticks into the molds.

4. Place the molds in the freezer and let the popsicles freeze completely, usually for about 4-6 hours or overnight.

5. Once frozen, remove the popsicles from the molds and enjoy.

Oven-Baked Sweet Potato Fries

Ingredients:

- 2 large sweet potatoes
- 2 tablespoons olive oil
- 1 teaspoon paprika
- 1/2 teaspoon garlic powder
- Salt and pepper, to taste

Instructions:

1. Preheat the oven to 425°F (220°C) and line a baking sheet with parchment paper.

2. Peel the sweet potatoes and cut them into thin strips resembling fries.

3. In a large bowl, toss the sweet potato strips with olive oil, paprika, garlic powder, salt, and pepper until well coated.

4. Spread the sweet potato strips evenly on the prepared baking sheet, making sure they are not overcrowded.

5. Bake for 20-25 minutes, flipping the fries halfway through, until they are crispy and golden brown.

6. Remove from the oven and let them cool slightly before serving.

Cucumber and Hummus Bites

Ingredients:

- English cucumber
- Hummus
- Cherry tomatoes, halved
- Fresh parsley or dill, for garnish (optional)

Instructions:

1. Slice the cucumber into thick rounds.

2. Using a spoon or a melon baller, scoop out a small indentation in the center of each cucumber round.

3. Fill each indentation with a dollop of hummus.

4. Top each cucumber and hummus bite with a halved cherry tomato.

5. Garnish with fresh parsley or dill, if desired.

6. Arrange the cucumber and hummus bites on a serving platter and serve.

Roasted Chickpeas with Chili and Lime

Ingredients:

- 1 can chickpeas, drained and rinsed
- 1 tablespoon olive oil
- 1 teaspoon chili powder
- 1/2 teaspoon cumin
- 1/2 teaspoon garlic powder
- Zest of 1 lime
- Salt, to taste

Instructions:

1. Preheat the oven to 400°F (200°C) and line a baking sheet with parchment paper.

2. Pat dry the rinsed chickpeas using a clean kitchen towel or paper towels.

3. In a bowl, toss the chickpeas with olive oil, chili powder, cumin, garlic powder, lime zest, and salt until evenly coated.

4. Spread the chickpeas in a single layer on the prepared baking sheet.

5. Roast in the preheated oven for about 25-30 minutes, shaking the pan occasionally, until the chickpeas are golden and crispy.

6. Remove from the oven and let them cool before serving.

Zucchini Chips with Garlic and Parmesan

Ingredients:

- 2 medium zucchinis
- 2 tablespoons olive oil
- 1/4 cup grated Parmesan cheese
- 1/2 teaspoon garlic powder
- Salt and pepper, to taste

Instructions:

1. Preheat the oven to 425°F (220°C) and line a baking sheet with parchment paper.

2. Slice the zucchinis into thin rounds.

3. In a bowl, toss the zucchini slices with olive oil, grated Parmesan cheese, garlic powder, salt, and pepper until well coated.

4. Arrange the zucchini slices in a single layer on the prepared baking sheet.

5. Bake for 15-20 minutes, flipping the slices halfway through, until the chips are crispy and lightly browned.

6. Remove from the oven and let them cool before serving.

Smoked Salmon Cucumber Rolls

Ingredients:

- English cucumber
- Smoked salmon slices
- Cream cheese
- Fresh dill, for garnish

Instructions:

1. Slice the cucumber lengthwise into thin strips using a mandoline or a vegetable peeler.

2. Pat the cucumber strips dry with a paper towel.

3. Spread a thin layer of cream cheese onto each
    cucumber strip.

4. Place a slice of smoked salmon onto the cream
    cheese-covered side of the cucumber strip.

5. Roll up the cucumber strip, securing the smoked
    salmon in the center.

6. Garnish with fresh dill and secure the rolls with
    toothpicks, if necessary.

7. Arrange the smoked salmon cucumber rolls on a
    serving platter and serve.

Turkey and Cheese Roll-Ups

Ingredients:

- Deli turkey slices
- Sliced cheese (cheddar, Swiss, or your choice)
- Mustard or mayonnaise, for spreading
- Lettuce leaves

Instructions:

1. Lay a slice of deli turkey flat on a clean surface.

2. Spread a thin layer of mustard or mayonnaise onto
    the turkey slice.

3. Place a slice of cheese on top of the spread.

4. Add a lettuce leaf on top of the cheese slice.

5. Roll up the turkey slice tightly, securing the ingredients within.

6. Repeat the process with the remaining turkey slices and ingredients.

7. Cut each rolled-up turkey slice into bite-sized pieces, if desired.

8. Arrange the turkey and cheese roll-ups on a serving platter and serve.

Edamame with Sea Salt

Ingredients:

- Frozen edamame
- Sea salt, to taste

Instructions:

1. Cook the frozen edamame according to the package instructions.

2. Once cooked, drain the edamame and transfer them to a bowl.

3. Sprinkle sea salt over the cooked edamame while
    they are still warm.

4. Toss the edamame gently to ensure they are evenly
    coated with salt.

5. Serve the edamame as a nutritious and satisfying
    snack.

Stuffed Mini Bell Peppers with Cream Cheese

Ingredients:

* Mini bell peppers, halved and seeds removed
* Cream cheese
* Chopped fresh herbs (such as parsley or chives), for garnish

Instructions:

1. Preheat the oven to 375°F (190°C) and line a baking
    sheet with parchment paper.

2. Fill each halved mini bell pepper with cream
    cheese, spreading it evenly.

3. Arrange the stuffed mini bell peppers on the
    prepared baking sheet.

4. Bake for about 15-20 minutes, until the peppers are tender and the cream cheese is slightly golden.

5. Remove from the oven and garnish with chopped fresh herbs.

6. Allow the stuffed mini bell peppers to cool slightly before serving.

Chapter 6: Desserts

Berry Chia Seed Jam

Ingredients:

- 2 cups mixed berries (strawberries, blueberries, raspberries)
- 2 tablespoons chia seeds
- 1 tablespoon lemon juice
- 2 tablespoons honey or your preferred sweetener (optional)

Instructions:

1. Wash the mixed berries thoroughly and remove any stems or leaves.
2. Place the berries in a saucepan and heat them over medium heat.
3. Mash the berries using a fork or potato masher until they reach your desired consistency.
4. Add chia seeds and lemon juice to the saucepan and stir well.

5. Cook the mixture for about 5 minutes, stirring occasionally.

6. Remove the saucepan from heat and let the jam cool.

7. If desired, add honey or your preferred sweetener and mix well.

8. Transfer the jam to a jar or container and refrigerate for at least 1 hour to allow it to thicken.

9. Enjoy the berry chia seed jam on toast, pancakes, or as a topping for yogurt.

Baked Apples with Cinnamon and Walnuts

Ingredients:

- 4 apples (any variety)
- 1/4 cup chopped walnuts
- 1 teaspoon ground cinnamon
- 2 tablespoons honey or maple syrup
- 2 tablespoons unsalted butter, melted

Instructions:

1. Preheat your oven to 375°F (190°C).

2. Wash the apples and remove the cores using an apple corer or a knife.

3. Place the apples in a baking dish.

4. In a small bowl, mix together the chopped walnuts, ground cinnamon, and honey (or maple syrup).

5. Fill the center of each apple with the walnut mixture.

6. Drizzle the melted butter over the apples.

7. Bake the apples in the preheated oven for 25-30 minutes or until they are tender.

8. Remove the baked apples from the oven and let them cool slightly before serving.

9. Serve the baked apples as they are or with a scoop of vanilla ice cream for an extra treat.

Chocolate Avocado Mousse

Ingredients:

- 2 ripe avocados
- 1/4 cup unsweetened cocoa powder
- 1/4 cup honey or your preferred sweetener
- 1 teaspoon vanilla extract
- Pinch of salt

- Optional toppings: shaved dark chocolate, sliced strawberries

Instructions:

1. Cut the avocados in half, remove the pits, and scoop the flesh into a blender or food processor.
2. Add cocoa powder, honey (or your preferred sweetener), vanilla extract, and a pinch of salt to the blender.
3. Blend the ingredients until smooth and creamy.
4. If the mixture is too thick, you can add a tablespoon of milk (dairy or plant-based) to thin it out.
5. Once blended, transfer the chocolate avocado mousse to serving dishes or glasses.
6. Refrigerate for at least 1 hour to chill and set.
7. Before serving, you can sprinkle some shaved dark chocolate or add sliced strawberries on top for garnish.
8. Enjoy the rich and creamy chocolate avocado mousse as a guilt-free dessert option.

Greek Yogurt and Mixed Berry Parfait

Ingredients:

- 1 cup Greek yogurt
- 1 cup mixed berries (strawberries, blueberries, raspberries)
- 1/4 cup granola
- 1 tablespoon honey or maple syrup (optional)

Instructions:

1. In a glass or jar, start by layering 1/4 cup of Greek yogurt at the bottom.
2. Add a layer of mixed berries on top of the yogurt.
3. Sprinkle a tablespoon of granola over the berries.
4. Repeat the layers until all the ingredients are used, ending with a layer of Greek yogurt on top.
5. If desired, drizzle honey or maple syrup over the top layer of Greek yogurt for added sweetness.
6. Refrigerate the parfait for 30 minutes to allow the flavors to meld together.

7. Serve the Greek yogurt and mixed berry parfait chilled as a refreshing and nutritious dessert or snack.

Sugar-Free Blueberry Cheesecake Bites

Ingredients:

- 1 cup fresh or frozen blueberries
- 1 cup cream cheese (regular or low-fat), softened
- 1/4 cup powdered erythritol or your preferred sugar substitute
- 1 teaspoon vanilla extract
- Fresh mint leaves for garnish (optional)

Instructions:

1. In a mixing bowl, combine the softened cream cheese, powdered erythritol (or your preferred sugar substitute), and vanilla extract. Mix until smooth and well combined.
2. Gently fold in the blueberries, being careful not to mash them.

3. Spoon the mixture into silicone molds or ice cube trays, filling each cavity.

4. Tap the molds lightly on the countertop to remove any air bubbles and smooth the surface.

5. Place the molds in the freezer and freeze for at least 2 hours or until the cheesecake bites are firm.

6. Once frozen, remove the cheesecake bites from the molds and transfer them to a container or freezer bag.

7. Store the bites in the freezer until ready to serve.

8. Before serving, let the blueberry cheesecake bites thaw for a few minutes.

9. Garnish with fresh mint leaves if desired and enjoy the guilt-free sweetness.

Almond Flour Chocolate Chip Cookies

Ingredients:

- 2 cups almond flour
- 1/4 cup coconut oil, melted
- 1/4 cup honey or maple syrup
- 1 teaspoon vanilla extract

- 1/2 teaspoon baking soda

- 1/4 teaspoon salt

- 1/2 cup sugar-free dark chocolate chips

Instructions:

1. Preheat your oven to 350°F (175°C) and line a baking sheet with parchment paper.

2. In a mixing bowl, combine the almond flour, melted coconut oil, honey (or maple syrup), vanilla extract, baking soda, and salt. Mix well until a dough forms.

3. Fold in the sugar-free dark chocolate chips until evenly distributed.

4. Scoop tablespoon-sized portions of dough onto the prepared baking sheet, spacing them apart.

5. Gently flatten each cookie with the back of a spoon or your palm.

6. Bake in the preheated oven for 10-12 minutes or until the edges turn golden brown.

7. Remove the cookies from the oven and let them cool on the baking sheet for a few minutes.

8. Transfer the almond flour chocolate chip cookies to a wire rack to cool completely before serving.

9. Enjoy these delightful, gluten-free cookies as a healthier alternative to traditional chocolate chip cookies.

Coconut and Lime Energy Balls

Ingredients:

- 1 cup unsweetened shredded coconut
- 1/2 cup almond flour
- 1/4 cup coconut oil, melted
- 2 tablespoons lime juice
- 2 tablespoons honey or maple syrup
- 1 teaspoon lime zest
- Pinch of salt

Instructions:

1. In a mixing bowl, combine the unsweetened shredded coconut, almond flour, melted coconut oil, lime juice, honey (or maple syrup), lime zest, and a pinch of salt.

2. Mix well until the ingredients are evenly combined and the mixture holds together when pressed.

3. Using your hands, shape the mixture into small bite-sized balls.

4. Place the coconut and lime energy balls on a baking sheet lined with parchment paper.

5. Refrigerate the energy balls for at least 1 hour to firm up.

6. Once chilled, transfer the energy balls to an airtight container and store them in the refrigerator.

7. Enjoy these refreshing and nutritious coconut and lime energy balls as a quick snack or a pick-me-up during the day.

Pumpkin Spice Chia Pudding

Ingredients:

- 1/4 cup chia seeds
- 1 cup unsweetened almond milk or your preferred milk
- 1/4 cup pumpkin puree
- 1 tablespoon maple syrup or your preferred sweetener
- 1/2 teaspoon pumpkin spice blend

- Optional toppings: chopped nuts, pumpkin seeds, cinnamon

Instructions:

1. In a bowl, combine the chia seeds, almond milk (or your preferred milk), pumpkin puree, maple syrup (or your preferred sweetener), and pumpkin spice blend.
2. Stir well to make sure all the ingredients are thoroughly mixed.
3. Let the mixture sit for 5 minutes, then stir again to prevent clumping of the chia seeds.
4. Cover the bowl and refrigerate the chia pudding for at least 2 hours or overnight.
5. Before serving, give the chia pudding a good stir to distribute the pumpkin puree evenly.
6. Spoon the pumpkin spice chia pudding into serving bowls or glasses.
7. Top with chopped nuts, pumpkin seeds, or a sprinkle of cinnamon, if desired.

8. Enjoy the creamy and flavorful pumpkin spice chia pudding as a satisfying dessert or even a breakfast option.

Peanut Butter and Banana Ice Cream

Ingredients:

- 3 ripe bananas, sliced and frozen
- 2 tablespoons natural peanut butter
- Optional toppings: crushed peanuts, dark chocolate chips

Instructions:

1. Place the frozen banana slices in a blender or food processor.
2. Add the peanut butter to the blender.
3. Blend the ingredients until smooth and creamy, scraping down the sides as needed.
4. If the mixture is too thick, you can add a tablespoon of milk (dairy or plant-based) to help with blending.
5. Transfer the peanut butter and banana mixture to a freezer-safe container.

6. Freeze the ice cream for at least 2 hours or until firm.

7. Once frozen, scoop the peanut butter and banana ice cream into bowls or cones.

8. Top with crushed peanuts or dark chocolate chips for added crunch and flavor, if desired.

9. Indulge in this simple and delightful peanut butter and banana ice cream, which is a healthier alternative to traditional ice cream.

Strawberry Frozen Yogurt Bark

Ingredients:

- 2 cups plain Greek yogurt
- 1 cup fresh strawberries, sliced
- 2 tablespoons honey or maple syrup
- 1/4 cup granola

Instructions:

1. Line a baking sheet with parchment paper.

2. In a bowl, mix together the Greek yogurt and honey (or maple syrup) until well combined.

3. Spread the Greek yogurt mixture evenly onto the prepared baking sheet.

4. Arrange the sliced strawberries on top of the yogurt.

5. Sprinkle the granola over the strawberries, pressing it lightly into the yogurt.

6. Place the baking sheet in the freezer and freeze for at least 2 hours or until the yogurt bark is firm.

7. Once frozen, remove the bark from the baking sheet and break it into smaller pieces.

8. Store the strawberry frozen yogurt bark in an airtight container in the freezer until ready to serve.

9. Enjoy the refreshing and fruity goodness of this homemade frozen yogurt bark as a cool treat.

Raspberry and Almond Flour Cake

Ingredients:

- 2 cups almond flour
- 1/4 cup coconut flour
- 1/4 cup granulated erythritol or your preferred sugar substitute
- 1 teaspoon baking powder
- 1/4 teaspoon salt

- 1/2 cup unsalted butter, melted
- 4 large eggs
- 1/4 cup unsweetened almond milk or your preferred milk
- 1 teaspoon vanilla extract
- 1 cup fresh raspberries

Instructions:

1. Preheat your oven to 350°F (175°C). Grease a round cake pan with butter or line it with parchment paper.
2. In a mixing bowl, combine the almond flour, coconut flour, granulated erythritol (or your preferred sugar substitute), baking powder, and salt.
3. In a separate bowl, whisk together the melted butter, eggs, almond milk (or your preferred milk), and vanilla extract.
4. Add the wet ingredients to the dry ingredients and stir until well combined.
5. Gently fold in the fresh raspberries.
6. Pour the batter into the prepared cake pan and spread it evenly.

7. Bake in the preheated oven for 25-30 minutes or until a toothpick inserted into the center comes out clean.

8. Remove the cake from the oven and let it cool in the pan for 10 minutes.

9. Transfer the raspberry and almond flour cake to a wire rack to cool completely before slicing and serving.

10. Enjoy a slice of this moist and flavorful cake as a delightful dessert or afternoon treat.

Chapter 7: Smoothies

Smoothies are a delightful and refreshing way to pack essential nutrients into your day. These smoothie recipes will not only tantalize your taste buds but also provide a nourishing boost to your body.

Green Detox Smoothie

Ingredients:

- 1 cup spinach leaves
- 1 ripe banana
- 1 small cucumber, peeled and chopped
- 1 celery stalk, chopped
- ½ lemon, juiced
- 1 teaspoon grated ginger
- ½ cup coconut water
- Ice cubes (optional)

Instructions:

1. Place all the ingredients in a blender.
2. Blend on high speed until smooth and creamy.

3. If desired, add ice cubes and blend again for a chilled smoothie.

4. Pour into a glass and enjoy this invigorating green detox smoothie.

Blueberry and Spinach Smoothie

Ingredients:

- 1 cup fresh or frozen blueberries
- 1 cup spinach leaves
- 1 ripe banana
- ½ cup Greek yogurt
- 1 tablespoon honey or maple syrup
- ½ cup almond milk

Instructions:

1. Add all the ingredients to a blender.

2. Blend until well combined and creamy.

3. Adjust the consistency by adding more almond milk if needed.

4. Pour into a glass and savor the sweet and tangy flavors of this blueberry and spinach smoothie.

Mango and Turmeric Smoothie

Ingredients:

- 1 ripe mango, peeled and pitted
- 1 medium-sized orange, peeled and segmented
- 1 teaspoon ground turmeric
- ½ cup coconut milk
- 1 tablespoon chia seeds
- 1 cup ice cubes

Instructions:

1. Place all the ingredients in a blender.
2. Blend until the mixture is smooth and creamy.
3. Add more coconut milk or water if a thinner consistency is desired.
4. Pour into a glass and enjoy the tropical goodness of this mango and turmeric smoothie.

Strawberry and Kale Smoothie

Ingredients:

- 1 cup fresh or frozen strawberries
- 1 cup kale leaves, stems removed
- 1 ripe banana

- ½ cup plain Greek yogurt
- 1 tablespoon honey or agave syrup
- ½ cup almond milk
- Ice cubes (optional)

Instructions:

1. Combine all the ingredients in a blender.
2. Blend until the mixture is smooth and velvety.
3. Add ice cubes if desired and blend again for a colder smoothie.
4. Pour into a glass and relish the delightful combination of strawberries and kale in this smoothie.

Avocado and Coconut Smoothie

Ingredients:

- ½ ripe avocado, pitted and peeled
- ½ cup coconut milk
- 1 ripe banana
- 1 tablespoon honey or maple syrup
- 1 tablespoon lime juice
- ½ cup spinach leaves

- ½ cup ice cubes

Instructions:

1. Add all the ingredients to a blender.
2. Blend until the mixture is creamy and well incorporated.
3. Adjust the sweetness with more honey or maple syrup if desired.
4. Pour into a glass and savor the creamy goodness of this avocado and coconut smoothie.

Pineapple and Ginger Smoothie

Ingredients:

- 1 cup fresh pineapple chunks
- 1 small banana
- ½ inch fresh ginger, peeled and grated
- ½ cup Greek yogurt
- 1 tablespoon honey or agave syrup
- ½ cup almond milk
- Ice cubes (optional)

Instructions:

1. Place all the ingredients in a blender.

2. Blend until the mixture is smooth and frothy.

3. If preferred, add ice cubes and blend again for a cooler smoothie.

4. Pour into a glass and enjoy the tropical tang of this pineapple and ginger smoothie.

Berry Blast Smoothie

Ingredients:

- 1 cup mixed berries (strawberries, raspberries, blueberries)
- ½ cup Greek yogurt
- 1 ripe banana
- 1 tablespoon honey or maple syrup
- ½ cup almond milk
- 1 tablespoon flaxseeds (optional)
- Ice cubes (optional)

Instructions:

1. Add all the ingredients to a blender.

2. Blend until the mixture is well combined and creamy.

3. Include flaxseeds for added fiber and omega-3 fatty acids if desired.

4. If a colder smoothie is preferred, add ice cubes and blend again.

5. Pour into a glass and relish the burst of berry flavors in this refreshing smoothie.

Peanut Butter and Banana Smoothie

Ingredients:

- 1 ripe banana
- 2 tablespoons natural peanut butter
- 1 cup almond milk
- 1 tablespoon honey or maple syrup
- ½ teaspoon vanilla extract
- ½ cup ice cubes

Instructions:

1. Place all the ingredients in a blender.

2. Blend until the mixture is smooth and creamy.

3. Adjust the sweetness with more honey or maple syrup if desired.

4. Add ice cubes and blend again for a frostier texture.

5. Pour into a glass and enjoy the delightful combination of peanut butter and banana in this smoothie.

Chocolate and Almond Smoothie

Ingredients:

- 1 ripe banana
- 2 tablespoons unsweetened cocoa powder
- 1 tablespoon almond butter
- 1 cup almond milk
- 1 tablespoon honey or maple syrup
- ½ teaspoon vanilla extract
- ½ cup ice cubes

Instructions:

1. Add all the ingredients to a blender.
2. Blend until the mixture is creamy and well blended.
3. Adjust the sweetness with more honey or maple syrup if desired.
4. Add ice cubes and blend again for a colder and thicker smoothie.

5. Pour into a glass and indulge in the luscious combination of chocolate and almond flavors.

Tropical Green Smoothie

Ingredients:

- 1 cup fresh or frozen pineapple chunks
- 1 cup fresh spinach leaves
- 1 ripe banana
- ½ cup coconut water
- 1 tablespoon chia seeds
- ½ cup ice cubes

Instructions:

1. Place all the ingredients in a blender.
2. Blend until the mixture is smooth and vibrant.
3. If desired, add more coconut water for a thinner consistency.
4. Add ice cubes and blend again for a cooler smoothie.
5. Pour into a glass and savor the tropical freshness of this green smoothie.

Coffee and Walnut Smoothie

Ingredients:

- 1 cup brewed coffee, chilled
- 1 ripe banana
- 2 tablespoons walnuts
- 1 tablespoon almond butter
- 1 tablespoon honey or maple syrup
- ½ cup almond milk
- ½ cup ice cubes

Instructions:

1. Add all the ingredients to a blender.
2. Blend until the mixture is smooth and creamy.
3. Adjust the sweetness with more honey or maple syrup if desired.
4. Include ice cubes for a frostier texture.
5. Pour into a glass and relish the invigorating blend of coffee and walnut in this smoothie.

CONCLUSION

Throughout this cookbook, we have strived to provide you with an extensive range of recipes that cover various meals and snacks, ensuring that your taste buds never grow bored. We have carefully curated an assortment of breakfast options, from savory omelets packed with nutritious vegetables to sweet and tangy overnight oats bursting with the flavors of cinnamon and apple. These breakfast recipes not only provide a delightful start to your day but also help stabilize blood sugar levels.

As we conclude this cookbook, we want to emphasize the importance of maintaining a healthy diabetic lifestyle beyond the 30-day plan. By embracing the principles of mindful eating, portion control, regular physical activity, and ongoing self-monitoring, you can continue to manage your diabetes effectively and enjoy a higher quality of life. Remember to consult with your healthcare provider or a registered dietitian for personalized advice and guidance tailored to your specific needs.

We sincerely hope that this 30-Day Diabetic Cookbook Meal Plan for Beginners has provided you with the tools, knowledge, and inspiration to embark on a delicious and fulfilling journey towards better health. We encourage you to experiment with the recipes, make them your own, and continue to explore new flavors and culinary possibilities.

We extend our deepest appreciation to the dedicated team of experts who contributed to the creation of this cookbook. Their passion, expertise, and commitment to promoting healthier lifestyles for individuals with diabetes have been invaluable.

Lastly, we would like to express our gratitude to you, the reader, for embarking on this culinary adventure with us. We hope that this cookbook has not only enlightened you about diabetes management but has also instilled a love for nutritious and flavorsome meals. Remember, every bite you take is an opportunity to nourish your body and savor the joy of a healthier life.